The Immunity Code

Discovering the Secrets to a Powerful and Durable Immune System

By

Mildred L. Washington

Copyright © by Mildred L. Washington 2023. All rights reserved.

Table of Content

Introduction

Our immune system is a wonderful and intricate kind of defense that shields us against a wide variety of dangerous infections and alien invaders. Its primary function is to ward off disease-causing microorganisms. Our immune system defends us against anything from bacteria and viruses to poisons and cancer cells, and this vital function is essential to maintaining our health and well-being.

Nonetheless, there are a number of things that might weaken or otherwise affect our immune system, making us more susceptible to illness and disease. Some of the things that can lower our resistance to illness include improper nutrition, a lack of sleep, high levels of stress, and contact with toxic substances in the environment.

The good news is that there are a number of things we can do to boost and enhance our immune system. These include engaging in regular physical activity, eating a healthy and balanced diet, getting adequate sleep, and effectively managing stress. We may enhance the natural defenses of our bodies and experience vigorous health throughout our entire lives if we take a holistic approach to caring for our health and well-being.

In this book, we will delve deeply into the science that underpins how our immune system operates and what we can do to support it. This will be an exciting journey into the intriguing world of immunity. We will go over the most recent findings from studies on immunity and its function in the prevention and treatment of a wide range of disorders. In addition, we will go over some practical ways to enhance our immune function and ensure that our health is at its best. This book is your guide to unlocking the power of immunity and achieving optimal health and vitality. Whether your goal is to improve your overall wellness, avoid or conquer specific health concerns, or both, you will find the information you need in this book.

Chapter 1

Introduction to Immunity

The capacity of an organism to withstand infection and sickness is what we mean when we talk about immunity. It is a vital component of the body's defense mechanisms against invading pathogens, including bacteria, viruses, and fungi. These infections can cause illness and even death in the body. As the intricate network of cells, tissues, and organs, the immune system's primary function is to identify and remove potentially hazardous chemicals from the body by working in concert with one another.

Both innate immunity and adaptive immunity are broad classifications that can be applied to the functions of the immune system. Innate immunity is the body's initial line of defense against invading pathogens, and it is constantly present and ready to respond to any threat. This immunity is the body's first line of defense against invading pathogens. It is made up of both physical barriers, such as the skin and mucous membranes, and a wide variety of cells and molecules that collaborate with one another to detect and eliminate harmful agents in a timely manner.

Adaptive immunity, on the other hand, is a response that is more specific and targeted, and it develops over time in response to exposure to particular infections. Adaptive immunity protects against diseases that are caused by specific pathogens. It involves the generation of antibodies, as well as specialized cells known as T cells and B cells, as well as a mechanism known as immunological memory, which enables the body to recall previous encounters with the same pathogen and react more quickly to subsequent encounters with the same agent.

The immune system is a highly advanced and intricate system that is essential to the body's ability to stay healthy and well. Its job is to protect the body from harmful pathogens. But, it is not foolproof, and there are occasions when it does not provide the body with sufficient protection against particular microorganisms, which can result in infections and disorders. It is, therefore, vital to have a solid understanding of the immune system and how it operates in order to develop effective therapies and prevention methods for a wide variety of diseases and illnesses.

An outline of the body's immune system

As the intricate network of cells, tissues, and organs, the immune system's primary function is to defend the body against potentially harmful pathogens, including bacteria, viruses, and fungi. This defense is provided by the immune system, which is a component of the immune system. It is an essential component of the body's defense processes since it helps to recognize and destroy aberrant cells and foreign substances, including cancer cells.

Innate immunity and adaptive immunity are the two primary classifications that can be used to describe the immune system. Innate immunity is the body's first line of defense, and it consists of both physical barriers, such as the skin and mucous membranes and a wide variety of cells and molecules that are able to identify and destroy invading pathogens. The skin is the body's largest organ and is responsible for protecting the body from the outside environment. Phagocytes (such as macrophages and neutrophils), natural killer cells, complement proteins, and cytokines are some examples of the cells and substances that fall under this category.

Adaptive immunity, also known as acquired immunity, is a type of immunity that develops through time in response to previous experiences with particular infections. It is a response that is more precise and targeted. It involves the generation of antibodies, as well as specialized cells known as T cells and B cells, as well as a mechanism known as immunological memory, which enables the body to recall previous encounters with the same pathogen and react more quickly to subsequent encounters with the same agent.

Antibodies are proteins that can identify and bind to certain foreign things, such as bacteria or viruses. B cells are the cells in the immune system that are responsible for making antibodies. T cells are the cells in the immune system that are in charge of immediately attacking and eliminating cells that have been infected with infections. T cells have the ability to help activate other immune cells, such as B cells and macrophages, which can then be used to assist in the battle against infections.

In addition, the immune system is comprised of a number of organs and tissues, such as the thymus, spleen, lymph nodes, and bone marrow. These organs and tissues are responsible for the production and storage of immune cells, as well as a significant part in the formation and control of the immune response. In general, the immune system is a complicated and highly developed system that plays an essential part in ensuring the body's continued health and well-being. It is vital for the development of effective therapies and preventative measures for a wide range of diseases and illnesses to have a better understanding of how the immune system operates. This information is essential.

Several distinct categories of immunological reactions

Innate immunity and adaptive immunity are the two primary types of responses that can be generated by the immune system. The body is protected from infections and other potentially hazardous substances because of the coordinated efforts of these reactions.

Immunity innate: The innate immune response is the body's initial line of defense against foreign pathogens that have invaded the body. It is a response that is not unique to any particular pathogen, yet it offers instant protection against a wide variety of infectious agents. The skin and mucous membranes are examples of physical barriers that are part of the innate immune system. Innate immunity also consists of a wide variety of cells and molecules that collaborate to quickly identify and eliminate harmful agents. The following are some of the most important aspects of the innate immune response:

Barriers of a physical nature, such as the mucous membranes and the skin

Phagocytes are white blood cells that consume and eliminate invading pathogens. Examples of phagocytes include macrophages and neutrophils.

Natural killer cells, often known as NK cells, are cells that eliminate infected or aberrant cells.

Complement proteins are responsible for the formation of pores in the membranes of pathogens, which ultimately results in the killing of the pathogens.

Cytokines, which help recruit other immune cells to the site of infection and govern the immunological response, are responsible for this.

Adaptive immunity: The adaptive immune response is a reaction that is more precise and focused than the innate immune response. It is a response that develops over time as a result of exposure to particular infections. It involves the generation of antibodies, as well as specialized cells known as T cells and B cells, as well as a mechanism known as immunological memory, which enables the body to recall previous encounters with the same pathogen and react more quickly to subsequent encounters with the same agent. The following are some of the most important aspects of the adaptive immune response:

B cells are responsible for the production of antibodies, which are able to identify and bind to particular foreign invaders, such as viruses and bacteria.

T cells are responsible for the direct assault and annihilation of cells that have been infected by pathogens.

Immunological memory, which enables the body to remember previous encounters with a pathogen and react more quickly to subsequent encounters with that infection

Both innate and adaptive immune responses are required for the body to successfully defend itself against infectious agents and to keep its general health in good standing. The development of effective therapies and prevention measures for a wide variety of diseases and illnesses can be aided by a greater knowledge of how these responses work.

Chapter 2

The Structure and Function of the Immune System's Anatomy and Physiology

An intricate network of cells, tissues, and organs, the immune system's primary function is to defend the body against invading microorganisms and other types of foreign substances that may be harmful. A brief summary of the immune system's anatomy and physiology can be found as follows:

The primary lymphoid organs are as follows:

Primary lymphoid organs are the places in the body that are responsible for the production and maturation of immune cells. Bone marrow and the thymus gland are both examples of these tissues. The bone marrow is responsible for the production and storage of stem cells, which can differentiate into many different types of immune cells, such as B cells, T cells, and natural killer cells. It is in the thymus gland that T cells complete their maturation and division into the several subsets of T cells that are responsible for the varied tasks of the immune system.

The activation of immune cells and the immunological response both take place in the secondary lymphoid organs, which can be thought of as the "secondary" part of the lymphoid system. Lymph nodes, the spleen, and mucosal-associated lymphoid tissue are all considered to be part of this system (MALT). The lymph nodes are responsible for filtering the lymphatic fluid and are also the location where immune cells become activated in response to the presence of foreign substances. The spleen is an important site for the development of immune responses against blood-borne infections because it filters blood and acts as a filter. The tonsils, adenoids, and Peyer patches in the gastrointestinal tract are all components of the MALT system, which is responsible for monitoring the mucosal surfaces of the body.

Cells of the immune system: The immune system is composed of a wide array of specialized cells that cooperate with one another to defend the body against foreign invaders. These are the following:

B cells: Antibodies are proteins that can recognize and bind to certain foreign things, such as bacteria or viruses. B cells are responsible for producing these antibodies. When B cells have been activated, they have the potential to develop into memory B cells, which enable the body to react more swiftly when it is exposed to the same pathogen again in the future.

T cells: T cells are responsible for directly attacking and eliminating cells that have been infected with pathogens. This is done via T cells' ability to recognize and target infected cells. They are also able to assist in the activation of other immune cells, such as B cells and macrophages, which can be of assistance in the battle against infections. T cells can be broken down into a number of distinct subsets, each of which serves a unique purpose in the body's immunological response.

Natural killer (NK) cells are specialized immune cells that are able to identify and eliminate aberrant or contaminated cells. NK cells are referred to as "killer" cells.

Molecules: The immune system relies on a variety of molecules to assist in recognizing and eliminating infections in the body. These are the following:

Antibodies are proteins that are created by B cells. They are able to recognize and bind to certain foreign objects, such as bacteria or viruses. Antibodies are produced by B cells. They have the ability to activate the complement system, which is a group of proteins that collaborate to eliminate harmful organisms. Cytokines are a type of signaling molecule that plays an important role in the regulation of the immune response as well as in the communication between immune cells.

Complement proteins are a group of proteins that eliminate harmful microorganisms by cooperating with one another. Complement proteins are also known as complement factors. They have the ability to create pores in the membranes of infections, which ultimately results in the demise of the pathogens.

In general, the immune system is a complicated and highly developed system that plays an essential part in ensuring the body's continued health and well-being. A greater understanding of its architecture and physiology can assist in the development of effective treatments and prevention measures for a wide variety of diseases and disorders. This can be a significant contribution.

Components of the immune system that are cellular and molecular in nature

The immune system is a complicated network of cells and molecules that cooperate to defend the body against potentially dangerous diseases and other invading substances. The following is an outline of some of the most important cellular and molecular components that make up the immune system:

Leukocytes:

White blood cells, often known as leukocytes, are the cells that make up the immune system. Granulocytes and agranulocytes are the two primary classifications that may be applied to them. Granulocytes are a type of leukocyte that have granules present in their cytoplasm. Granulocytes are also known as macrophages. These white blood cells consist of neutrophils, basophils, and eosinophils. Neutrophils are the most common form of granulocyte, and their function in the body's innate immune response is essential. Both eosinophils and basophils play a role in the immune response, although eosinophils are more important in the fight against allergic reactions.

Agranulocytes are a type of leukocyte that do not have granules present in their cytoplasm. Agranulocytes are also known as neutrophils. Lymphocytes and monocytes are included in this group. Lymphocytes are cells that are involved in the innate immune response as well as the adaptive immunological response. Lymphocytes comprise B cells, T cells, and natural killer (NK) cells. The activation of the adaptive immune response is dependent on monocytes undergoing differentiation into dendritic cells and macrophages, both of which are critical components of the innate immune response.

Antibodies: Antibodies, also known as immunoglobulins, are proteins produced by B cells that recognize and bind to certain foreign things, such as bacteria or viruses. Antibodies are also known as immunoglobulins. Antibodies are able to activate the complement system, which is comprised of a series of proteins that collaborate to eliminate infections. The complement system: The complement system is comprised of a number of proteins that collaborate to eliminate pathogens. It is able to create pores in the membranes of infections, which ultimately results in the demise of the pathogens. Antibodies are necessary for the activation of the complement system, but some chemicals that are produced by other immune cells are also necessary. Cytokines are a type of signaling molecule that plays an important role in the regulation of the immune response as well as in the communication between immune cells. They are able to be generated by a wide variety of cell types, including T cells, B cells, macrophages, and dendritic cells, among others. Cytokines are capable of stimulating inflammation, activating immune cells, and controlling the adaptive immune response, all of which are examples of the vast range of impacts that they can have on immune cells.

Toll-like receptors are as follows:

Toll-like receptors are a particular kind of receptor that may be discovered on the surface of various immune cells. They are able to identify certain chemicals that are linked with pathogens, such as components of the bacterial cell wall or viral nucleic acids. Toll-like receptors have the ability to activate immune cells and play an important role in the initiation of an immunological response.

To summarize, in order to defend the body against pathogens and other external substances, the cellular and molecular components of the immune system collaborate in a manner that is intricate and well-coordinated with one another. The creation of successful therapies and preventative measures for a wide variety of diseases and illnesses can be aided by a greater understanding of these components, which can be helpful in the development of such treatments and strategies.

Those parts of the body are responsible for immune function. The immune system is comprised of many different organs and tissues located all over the body, in addition to the cellular and molecular components.

The following is a list of important organs and tissues that have a role in immunity:

The soft, sponge-like tissue that can be discovered inside bones is referred to as "bone marrow." It is in charge of the generation of all of the different types of blood cells, including leukocytes, which are the cells that make up the immune system.

One of the glands that can be found in the chest, directly above the heart, is called the thymus. It is in charge of the maturation and differentiation of T cells, which are a kind of lymphocyte engaged in the adaptive immune response. T cells are matured and differentiated by this factor.

The spleen is an organ that can be found in the upper left quadrant of the abdominal cavity. It plays a role in the process of filtering the blood and eliminating damaged or aging red blood cells. Also containing immune cells and playing a vital role in the beginning stages of the immune response is the spleen.

Lymph nodes are bean-shaped structures that can be found all over the body. Lymph nodes are quite small. They are in charge of filtering out and entrapping foreign things, including bacteria or viruses and kicking off an immunological response in the body.

Mucosal tissues: Mucosal tissues are found in sections of the body that are exposed to the external environment, such as the respiratory system, the gastrointestinal tract, and the urogenital tract. Mucosal tissues protect these areas of the body from infection and disease. They guard against infections at these places thanks to the specific immune cells that they contain, such as mucosa-associated lymphoid tissue (MALT), which is an important example.

The skin is the body's biggest organ and a vital barrier against infection. It also plays a role in regulating body temperature. It is composed of immunological cells, including dendritic cells and Langerhans cells, which play a role in both innate and adaptive immune responses.

Gut-associated lymphoid tissue, also known as GALT, is a specific type of tissue that may be found in the gut. It is composed of immune cells and contains Peyer's patches and mesenteric lymph nodes, among other things. It has an important role in preventing infections in the gastrointestinal system where it is present.

The function of the immune system as a whole is to defend the body against potentially harmful infections and other external substances through the coordinated efforts of its organs and tissues. The immune response is initiated and coordinated in a variety of ways, each of which is dependent on a specific component. When it comes to immunity, having a solid understanding of the roles that various organs and tissues play can be of great assistance in the creation of novel treatments and preventative measures for a wide variety of diseases and illnesses.

Interactions between the physiological systems of the body, including the immune system

The immune system is intricately connected to the body's other physiological systems, making it difficult to separate the two. The following is a list of instances of interactions that can occur between the immune system and other systems:

The neurological system is able to exert some control over the immune response by means of the neurotransmitters and neuropeptides that it secretes. For instance, stress can result in the release of the hormone cortisol, which has the ability to dampen the immunological response. In addition, the immune system has the ability to secrete cytokines, which are molecules that are able to communicate with the neural system and regulate mood as well as behavior.

The release of hormones by the endocrine system helps to regulate the immune response. The endocrine system is engaged in the regulation of the immunological response. For instance, the thymus gland generates hormones that regulate the maturation of T lymphocytes, whereas the adrenal gland produces cortisol, which can have immunosuppressive effects on the body. Both of these glands are located in the chest.

The respiratory system is a potential entry point for infectious agents, making the immune system a crucial component in the process of defending the lungs and airways against bacterial, viral, and fungal diseases. In addition, the respiratory system is home to specialized immune cells, such as alveolar macrophages and dendritic cells, which play an essential role in the activation of the immune system in response to respiratory infections.

The gastrointestinal system is the location of billions of bacteria, which collectively are referred to as the gut microbiota. These bacteria have the ability to communicate with the immune system. Disturbances in the microbiota of the gut have been linked to a wide variety of diseases, including autoimmune disorders and infections, which suggests that the gut microbiota may play a role in the regulation of the immune response.

Cardiovascular system: Inflammation, a fundamental aspect of the immune response, is capable of having a negative impact on the cardiovascular system. Inflammation that is present for a longer period of time has been linked to the development of cardiovascular disorders, including atherosclerosis.

The immune system plays a significant function in the control and regulation of the reproductive system of females, particularly during pregnancy. This is especially true of the female reproductive system. The immune system, in addition to its other functions, is involved in the process of warding off sexually transmitted diseases.

In general, the immune system is not a stand-alone system; rather, it is tightly integrated with a variety of other physiological systems throughout the body. The better we understand these connections, the more likely it is that we will be able to develop effective therapies and preventative measures for a wider variety of diseases and disorders.

Chapter 3

Innate Immunity

The initial line of defense against invading viruses and other foreign substances is a person's innate immunity. It is the body's immediate, non-specific response to a threat, such as an illness or damage, and it is present from birth onward. The protection afforded by innate immunity is very instantaneous; nevertheless, it is not specific to any one particular pathogen and cannot, unlike adaptive immunity, offer protection that is maintained over time. The following is a list of some of the most important aspects of innate immunity:

1. Obstacles of a physical and chemical nature: Infectious agents are unable to enter the body because it is protected by a number of physical barriers. They include the skin and the mucous membranes. Chemical barriers, such as antimicrobial peptides and enzymes found in tears and saliva, have the ability to either eradicate bacteria entirely or slow down their rate of multiplication.

2. Phagocytes: Phagocytes are specialized cells that have the ability to ingest invading pathogens and then destroy them. There are two different kinds of phagocytes: neutrophils and macrophages. Neutrophils are the most common type of white blood cell and are involved in the initial stages of the immune response. Macrophages are larger and have a longer lifespan than neutrophils. Macrophages are involved in the later stages of the immune response.

3. Natural killer cells, also known as NK cells, are a subset of lymphocytes that have the ability to identify and eliminate malignant or contaminated cells. They are able to accomplish this goal by releasing poisonous chemicals that trigger the process of planned cell death known as apoptosis.

4. The complement system is a collection of proteins that can become active in response to an injury or an infection. The activated complement proteins have the ability to eliminate pathogens directly, attract phagocytes to the site of infection, and trigger the release of inflammatory chemicals.

5. Cytokines: Cytokines are molecules of signaling that are produced by immune cells. They have a role in the control of the immune response and are produced by immune cells. They have the ability to increase inflammation, encourage the generation of additional immune cells, and assist in the coordination of the responses of various immune cells.

The more specific adaptive immunity takes time to develop, while innate immunity is present at birth and provides rapid protection against infections. Innate immunity is an essential component of the immune system. The different aspects of innate immunity cooperate with one another to recognize and eliminate invading pathogens, as well as to set off an inflammatory response that can assist in the process of eliminating infections.

The first lines of protection that the body has against infectious agents are its physical and chemical barriers. These barriers, which are crucial components of the body's innate immune system, prohibit infections from entering the body and serve to keep the body healthy.

The following is a list of instances of both chemical and physical barriers to infection:

1. The skin: The skin serves as the body's initial line of protection against any diseases that may enter. It is a physical barrier that keeps pathogens from entering the body and doing their damage there. In addition to sweat, the skin produces sebum, an oily material that inhibits the growth of microorganisms like bacteria and fungi.

2. Mucous membranes: Mucous membranes are found in sections of the body that are exposed to the outside environment, such as the respiratory, gastrointestinal, and genitourinary systems. These areas include the genitourinary tract, the digestive tract, and the urinary tract. These membranes secrete mucus, which ensnares infectious agents and stops them from entering the body where they can do their damage. Mucous membranes are also responsible for the production of enzymes and antibodies, both of which can eliminate infections.

3. Cilia: The structures that look like hair and line the respiratory tract are called cilia. They work in unison to clear mucus and any infections that have become lodged in the respiratory tract.

4. Tears: Tears include enzymes and antibodies in them that can kill bacteria and viruses. The act of blinking helps to distribute tears around the surface of the eye, which washes away any infections that may have made their way into the eye.

5. Saliva: Saliva includes enzymes that have the ability to break down the cell walls of germs, hence inhibiting the growth of bacteria.

6. The acid produced by the stomach: Hydrochloric acid, which is produced by the stomach, has the ability to kill many different types of bacteria and viruses that enter the digestive tract.

7. The flow of urine: The movement of urine through the urinary tract helps to rid the body of any infections that may have been introduced into the body.

These physical and chemical barriers are essential components of the innate immune system, and they serve as the body's initial line of defense against infectious diseases. In the event that viruses are able to circumvent these defenses, the innate immune system is equipped with additional defenses to assist in the fight against the

infection. These defenses include phagocytes, natural killer cells, and the complement system.

The various biological components that make up an individual's innate immune system include several types of cells that are able to identify pathogens, damaged cells, or foreign substances and react appropriately to them.

The following is a list of some instances of cellular components that are involved in innate immunity:

1. Neutrophils: Neutrophils are the most common form of white blood cell and are the first cells to arrive at the site of an infection. Neutrophils also play an important role in the immune system. They are able to identify and consume a wide variety of pathogens, including bacteria, fungi, and others.

2. Macrophages: Macrophages are cells that play a role in the later phases of the immune response. These cells are larger and have a longer lifespan than other immune cells. They are able to identify and engulf a wide variety of pathogens, and they also have the ability to deliver antigens to T cells, which assists in the activation of the adaptive immune response.

3. Dendritic cells: Dendritic cells are specialized cells that can acquire antigens and present them to T cells, which helps to trigger the adaptive immune response. Dendritic cells have been shown to play an important role in the immune system. These can be found in the tissues of the body that come into direct touch with the outside environment, such as the mucous membranes and the skin.

4. Natural killer cells, also known as NK cells, are a subset of lymphocytes that have the ability to identify and eliminate malignant or contaminated cells. They are able to accomplish this goal by releasing poisonous chemicals that trigger the process of planned cell death known as apoptosis.

5. Mast cells: Mast cells are found in tissues that are in contacts with the outside environment, such as the skin and mucous membranes. Mast cells are responsible for the body's immune response to foreign substances. In reaction to an infection or injury, these cells will release histamine as well as other pro-inflammatory chemicals.

6. Eosinophils: Eosinophils are engaged in response to parasites and can also play a function in allergic reactions. Eosinophils can also play a part in the immune system's response to allergens.

7. Basophils: Basophils are immune cells that function similarly to mast cells and are involved in the body's response to allergic reactions and infections caused by parasites.

These cellular components collaborate with one another to identify infections and other foreign substances and to respond appropriately to them. They are also capable of kicking off the inflammatory response, which is a critical component of the innate immune response. Inflammation not only draws immune cells to the location of an infection, but it also has the potential to stop the infection from spreading to other areas of the body.

Chapter 4

Immune Disorders and Diseases

The immune system is a very intricate network consisting of cells, tissues, and organs cooperating to defend the body against infections and other harmful agents. On the other hand, the immune system can occasionally fail, which can result in a wide variety of immunological-related disorders and diseases. The following are some instances of diseases and disorders related to the immune system:

Autoimmune diseases:

Autoimmune disorders are caused when the immune system of the body mistakenly assaults the body's own cells and tissues, thinking that they are foreign invaders. Diseases such as rheumatoid arthritis, multiple sclerosis, and lupus are all examples of autoimmune disorders.

Immunodeficiency disorders: Immunodeficiency illnesses manifest themselves when an individual's immune system is unable to defend the body against pathogens in an adequate manner. Primary immunodeficiency diseases, such as severe combined immunodeficiency (SCID) and acquired immunodeficiency syndrome (AIDS), are caused by the human immunodeficiency virus and are both examples of immunodeficiency disorders. The human immunodeficiency virus is also the source of AIDS (HIV).

Allergies are caused when the immune system inappropriately reacts to normally harmless things like pollen or dust mites, as in the case of pollen or dust allergies. The immune system reacts to allergens by producing an allergic response, which can result in symptoms such as hives, sneezing, and trouble breathing.

Diseases that are caused by inflammation: Diseases that are caused by inflammation develop when the immune system produces an inflammatory response that causes harm to healthy tissues. Psoriasis, asthma and inflammatory bowel disease (IBD) are all examples of disorders that fall within the category of inflammatory diseases.

Cancer: The immune system plays a significant part in the process of detecting and eliminating cancer cells in the body. On the other hand, cancer cells can occasionally escape detection by the immune system, which can result in the development of cancer.

Reactions known as hypersensitivity occur when the immune system overreacts to particular substances, such as medications or food. Hypersensitivity reactions can be life-threatening. These reactions can range from being somewhat harmless to extremely dangerous and, in some instances, can even be fatal. These are only a few instances of disorders and diseases related to the immune system. New treatments are continually being created in order to improve the quality of life of people who are afflicted with immunological disorders and diseases. This is an active area of research, as is the understanding of the mechanisms that are at the root of these diseases.

Autoimmune disorders

Autoimmune diseases are a collection of conditions in which the immune system mistakenly assaults and damages the body's own tissues. Autoimmune illnesses affect a wide variety of organs and systems. In healthy individuals, the immune system is able to tell the difference between "self" cells and "non-self" cells. But, in individuals with autoimmune illnesses, the immune system is unable to make this distinction, which results in an immune response directed against the body's own tissues. Autoimmune illnesses are those that attack the body's immune system and can have a wide range of effects, both in terms of symptoms and problems.

There are about 80 distinct types of autoimmune disorders. However, the following are some of the most frequent ones: Rheumatoid arthritis, also known as Rheumatoid arthritis, is a chronic inflammatory illness that affects the joints and can cause pain, swelling, and stiffness. It is one of the most common forms of autoimmune arthritis.

Lupus is a chronic autoimmune condition that can impact a variety of organs and tissues, including the skin, joints, and kidneys, amongst others.

Diabetes type 1: Diabetes type 1 is a chronic autoimmune condition that damages the pancreas. As a result of this disorder, the pancreas is unable to make insulin, which is required in order to maintain normal levels of blood sugar.

Multiple sclerosis is a chronic autoimmune condition that affects the nervous system and causes destruction to the myelin sheath that covers nerve cells. Multiple sclerosis is also known as MS.

Celiac disease is an autoimmune ailment that causes the immune system to attack the small intestine in response to gluten. Gluten is a protein that can be found in grains like wheat, barley, and rye.

Psoriasis is a persistent autoimmune illness that affects the skin, generating thick, scaly areas that can be irritating and painful. Psoriasis is characterized by a red, flaky appearance on the skin.

Hashimoto's thyroiditis is a kind of hypothyroidism that is caused by an autoimmune ailment known as Hashimoto's thyroiditis. This condition causes the immune system to target the thyroid gland.

There is still a lot of mystery surrounding autoimmune disorders, but it is generally accepted that they are brought on by a confluence of hereditary and environmental risk factors.

Medications that suppress the immune system are often part of the treatment plan for autoimmune illnesses. Alterations to one's lifestyle can also be helpful in the management of symptoms and the prevention of consequences.

Immunodeficiencies

Immunodeficiencies are a collection of conditions in which the immune system is unable to protect the body from infections and other dangers as efficiently as it normally would. Immunodeficiencies can be primary or acquired.

Genetic illnesses that are evident at birth and are caused by abnormalities in one or more components of the immune system are known as primary immunodeficiencies. There are around 400 major immunodeficiencies that are now understood, and each of these conditions can have an effect on a different component of the immune system, such as B cells, T cells, or phagocytes. Primary immunodeficiencies include conditions such as severe combined immunodeficiency (also known as SCID), X-linked agammaglobulinemia (also known as XLA), and common variable immunodeficiency (CVID).

On the other hand, causes like infections, drugs, or other medical conditions can lead to acquired immunodeficiencies.

These deficiencies can occur at any age. Acquired immunodeficiency syndrome, also known as AIDS, is the most well-known kind of acquired immunodeficiency. This condition is brought on by the human immunodeficiency virus (HIV). Other forms of acquired immunodeficiency include those that result after the administration of chemotherapy or radiation therapy, as well as certain autoimmune illnesses.

Immunodeficiencies can result in a wide variety of symptoms, some of which include persistent diarrhea, frequent and severe infections, and a delay in the healing process of wounds. The treatment for immunodeficiencies varies widely depending on the underlying cause of the condition. Potential treatments for immunodeficiencies include immunoglobulin replacement therapy, antibiotics to treat infections, and drugs that stimulate the immune system.

Those who are immunocompromised are at a greater risk of contracting infections and experiencing other consequences; therefore, it is critical that they receive treatment and diagnosis as soon as possible. Genetic counseling is another treatment option that may be suggested to patients and their families who have primary immune weaknesses.

Reactions caused by allergies and other types of hypersensitivity

Both allergies and hypersensitivity reactions are immunological responses that are triggered by innocuous items in the environment, such as pollen, dust, or particular foods. Allergies and hypersensitivity reactions can be life-threatening. In people who have allergies, the immune system reacts excessively to these substances and produces a response that can cause a wide variety of symptoms. Some of these symptoms include rashes, sneezing, itching, and difficulty breathing.

On the basis of the type of immunological response that is manifested, allergies can be divided into the following four primary categories:

Type 1 hypersensitivity, also known as acute hypersensitivity, is the kind of allergy that affects most people and is also the most prevalent. Inflammation and other symptoms are brought on as a result of the activation of a specific type of immune cell known as a mast cell. Mast cells are responsible for the production of substances such as histamine. Allergic rhinitis, sometimes known as hay fever, is one example of a type 1 hypersensitivity reaction. Other examples include asthma and anaphylaxis. This particular form of hypersensitivity is known as type 2 hypersensitivity, and it is characterized by the development of antibodies that attack particular cells or tissues located within the body. The autoimmune form of hemolytic anemia and the drug-induced form of the condition are both examples of type 2 hypersensitivity reactions.

Type 3 hypersensitivity refers to the production of immune complexes, which are clusters of antibodies and antigens that can deposit themselves in tissues and produce inflammation. This type of hypersensitivity is characterized by the presence of immune complexes. Serum sickness and systemic lupus erythematosus are two examples of hypersensitivity reactions that fall into the type 3 category.

Type 4 hypersensitivity is also known as delayed-type hypersensitivity. It is characterized by the activation of certain immune cells known as T cells, which can lead to the destruction of tissue. Dermatitis caused by touch and various adverse reactions to medication is examples of type 4 hypersensitivity reactions.

The history of a patient's medical condition, a physical exam, and allergy testing (which may include skin tests and blood tests) are often the components that make up the diagnostic process for allergic reactions and hypersensitive reactions. Immunotherapy is used in severe cases to desensitize the immune system to the allergen that is causing the allergy or hypersensitivity reaction. Treatment for allergies and hypersensitivity reactions typically involves avoiding the allergen or substance that is causing the reaction, if this is possible.

Cancer and the body's defense mechanisms

The body's immune system is critically vital in the process of detecting and destroying cancer cells throughout the body. Cancer cells are aberrant cells that have the ability to expand and divide without being controlled, which may result in the development of tumors or other forms of cancer. On the other hand, the immune system is often able to recognize and destroy these cells before they become an issue for the body.

The immune system is able to identify and destroy cancer cells in a number of different ways, including the following:

Natural killer (NK) cells: There is a subset of immune cells known as natural killer cells (NK cells) that are able to directly identify and kill cancer cells without the necessity of previous sensitization.

T cells: T cells have the ability to recognize and kill cancer cells as well; however, they must first be sensitized to the cancer cells in order to do so. Lymphocytes that infiltrate tumors and are specific to cancer cells are called tumor-infiltrating lymphocytes (TILs).

Macrophages: Macrophages are immune cells that can ingest cancer cells and destroy them, as well as produce compounds that boost the immune response. Macrophages also play a role in the formation of antibodies.

On the other hand, there are instances in which cancer cells are able to elude the immune system and continue their growth and division despite being exposed. This can occur in a number of different ways, including the production of chemicals that inhibit the immune response or mutations that allow them to elude detection by the immune system. Both of these methods are examples of how this might take place.

Immunotherapy is a sort of treatment for cancer that works by inducing the body's immune system to identify and destroy cancer cells. There are many subsets of immunotherapy, such as monoclonal antibodies, checkpoint inhibitors, and adoptive cell transfer, among others. Some medicines have shown promise in combating some forms of cancer, but they are not successful against other types of the disease.

Other cancer treatments, such as chemotherapy and radiation therapy, can also have an effect on a patient's immune system. Immunotherapy is just one of these treatments. Because of these therapies, the number of immune cells that are found in the body can decrease, which makes it more difficult for the immune system to fend against infections and other types of danger. Yet, these treatments have the potential to stimulate the immune system, which in turn can assist in the elimination of cancer cells.

Chapter 5
Immunity and Health

Immunity is an extremely important factor in the preservation of overall health as well as the protection of the body from infectious diseases and other dangers. A robust immune system is one that is able to recognize and destroy malignant infections and aberrant cells while at the same time preventing an exaggerated response to non-threatening chemicals and the development of autoimmune or hypersensitive conditions. There are a number of factors, including the following, that have the potential to influence immunological function and general health.

Nutrition: Consuming the appropriate amount of key nutrients, such as vitamins and minerals, is necessary in order to keep one's immune system in good health. Malnutrition, on the other hand, is known to suppress the immune system and heighten a person's risk of contracting infectious diseases.

Exercising: Engaging in regular physical activity has been shown to improve immune function in a number of ways, including enhancing circulation, decreasing inflammation, and encouraging the generation of immune cells. [citation needed]

Sleep: Getting an adequate amount of sleep is critical to maintaining a healthy body and strong immune function. A lack of sleep can interfere with the immune system's regular functioning, which in turn can raise the likelihood of developing infections and other health issues.

The presence of persistent stress can have a detrimental impact on immune function and raise the likelihood of contracting infections as well as other health issues.

Environment: Being exposed to pollutants and poisons in the environment can have a negative impact on one's immune system, making them more likely to contract infections and have other negative health effects.

A healthy lifestyle that includes maintaining a balanced diet, engaging in regular physical activity, getting an adequate amount of sleep, and learning how to effectively manage stress can assist in boosting immune function and enhancing overall health. Moreover, vaccination and other preventative measures can assist in protecting against particular infectious diseases while also lowering the overall strain placed on the immune system.

Keeping an immune system that is in good shape

It is essential for one's general health and well-being to ensure that their immune system is in good shape. The following are some methods that you can maintain a healthy immune system and support the function of your immune system:

Eat a diet that is balanced: Essential nutrients that help the immune system can be obtained through the consumption of a diet that is abundant in fruits, vegetables, whole grains, lean proteins, and healthy fats. In addition to this, eating foods like berries, leafy greens, and nuts that are rich in antioxidants can aid in the reduction of inflammation and oxidative stress.

Exercise regularly: Frequent physical activity can increase immune function by boosting the generation of immune cells and lowering inflammation. This can be accomplished by exercising regularly. Your goal should be to get at least 150 minutes of moderate exercise or 75 minutes of strenuous exercise per week.

Obtain adequate rest. Having an adequate amount of sleep is critical for maintaining healthy immunological function as well as general health. Strive for seven to eight hours of sleep each night, and develop a regular sleep routine, to assist in the regulation of the clock that is found inside your body.

Take care of yourself: The immune system can be compromised by persistent stress, which also raises the likelihood of contracting infections and other health issues. Meditation, yoga, and other stress-relieving practices such as deep breathing exercises, should be practiced regularly.

It is important to refrain from smoking and drinking excessive amounts of alcohol because both of these habits can lower the body's immunological defenses, hence increasing the likelihood of contracting infections and other health issues.

Keep proper hygiene: It is possible to lower one's chance of contracting an illness by adhering to proper hygiene practices. These include frequently washing one's hands and avoiding contact with sick people.

Vaccinations can assist in guarding against certain infectious diseases and lower the overall burden that some diseases place on the immune system. Vaccinations should be kept up to date. You may help support the function of your immune system and contribute to the maintenance of a healthy immune system by implementing these healthy practices into your lifestyle.

The impact that nutrition and exercise have on a person's immunity

The immune system can be significantly influenced by both diet and physical activity levels. How to do it:

Diet: Essential nutrients that are required for proper immune function can be obtained through ingesting a diet that is rich in fruits, vegetables, whole grains, lean proteins, and healthy fats. Citrus fruits, fatty fish, nuts, and seeds, for instance, are good sources of vitamins C, D, zinc, and selenium, all of which are essential for proper immune system function and may be found in these foods. On the other side, a diet that is high in processed foods, added sugars, and saturated fats can contribute to chronic inflammation, which can impair the immune system. This is because processed foods and added sugars are both inflammatory. A poor diet can lead to obesity, which has been related to reduced immune function; obesity can also be the outcome of an unhealthy diet.

Exercise: Participating in regular physical exercise can increase the generation of immune cells and decrease inflammation, both of which can promote the operation of the immune system. In addition, physical activity can help reduce stress, which is known to inhibit immunological function. On the other hand, it is essential to keep in mind that engaging in an excessive amount of physical activity, such as endurance training or overtraining, might have the opposite impact and decrease immune function. As a result, it is essential to strike a balance and participate in an amount of exercise that is suitable for your current level of physical fitness.

In general, consuming a nutritious diet and engaging in regular physical activity can assist in supporting immune function and contribute to the maintenance of a healthy immune system. You can help to reduce inflammation, improve immune function, and support overall health and well-being by including a range of nutrient-dense foods in your diet and engaging in regular physical activity. If you do this, you will also be able to promote overall health and well-being.

Anxiety and the immune system

The immune system can be adversely affected by stress in a substantial way. The "fight or flight" reaction in the body is triggered whenever we are under emotional duress. This can momentarily lead to an increase in immune function. On the other hand, chronic stress, or stress that lasts for an extended length of time, can have the opposite impact and inhibit immune function. Chronic stress is defined as stress that lasts for an extended period of time.

The overproduction of stress hormones like cortisol, which can impair immune function by decreasing the production of immune cells and reducing the activity of immune cells that are already present, can be caused by chronic stress. Because of this, we may be more likely to contract infections and experience other health issues. Persistent stress can also contribute to chronic inflammation, which can further impair the immune system and raise the risk of infection. Chronic inflammation can also be a result of chronic stress.

Aside from that, stress can also have an effect on our behaviors and routines, such as the way we eat, how much we sleep, and how often we exercise. Chronic stress, for instance, has been linked to decreased quality and length of sleep, both of which might have an impact on immunological function. Overeating or undereating, both of which can contribute to inflammation and weaken the immune system, is another potential consequence of this condition. Last but not least, chronic stress can result in less time spent being physically active, which can also have a negative impact on immunological function.

It is imperative to engage in stress-reduction practices such as yoga, mindfulness meditation, and deep breathing exercises in order to not only boost immune function but also lessen the negative impact that stress has on the immune system. It is also essential to form healthy habits and routines, such as participating in regular physical activity, eating a portion of food that is balanced, and getting adequate sleep. We can contribute to the maintenance of a healthy immune system and minimize the risk of infections and other health problems if we take measures to manage stress and support the operation of the immune system.

Aging and immunity

The process of aging can have a major impact on immunological function, which can lead to an increased risk of developing infections and other health issues. The following is a list of the ways that getting older might impair one's immune system: Immunosenescence is a word that has been used to characterize the normal and inevitable reduction in the immunological function that comes with advancing age. As we get older, our immune systems become less effective at fighting off infections and producing immune cells. This is a natural consequence of aging. This may also increase the risk of autoimmune illnesses and cancer in addition to the danger of infections.

Inflammation that persists over time: Persistent low-grade inflammation, commonly referred to as "inflammaging," is a characteristic that is frequently associated with the aging process. This can lead to the development of chronic diseases, and it can also weaken the immune system, leaving us more susceptible to infections.

Alterations in the microbiome of the gut: The operation of the immune system is significantly impacted by the gut microbiome, which refers to the community of bacteria and other types of microbes that reside in our digestive tract. Changes in the composition of the gut microbiome that occur naturally with aging can have an effect on immune function and the likelihood of contracting infections.

Involution of the thymus: The thymus is the organ that is responsible for the production of T cells. T cells are a type of immune cell that plays an important role in the process of warding off infections. The thymus begins to atrophy as we get older, which can result in a decrease in the generation of T cells and a dysfunctional immune system.

It is essential for individuals who are getting older to engage in healthy habits such as regular physical activity, a balanced diet, and appropriate sleep in order to support the operation of their immune systems. In addition, vaccination against infectious diseases and regular checkups with a healthcare professional to evaluate the immune function and address any potential health issues that may occur can be beneficial for adults who are getting on in years.

Chapter 6

Immunology Future Directions

The science of immunology is one that is continuously undergoing new developments, and there are a number of fascinating areas of research that show promise for the development of immune-related treatments and therapies in the future. The following is a list of some of the current and upcoming study fields in the field of immunology: Immunotherapy in the treatment of cancer: Immunotherapy is a form of cancer treatment that works by directing the body's own immune system against the malignant cells that are responsible for the disease. There are many different kinds of immunotherapy, such as cancer vaccines and checkpoint inhibitors. CAR-T cell treatment is another sort of immunotherapy. Immunotherapy has been demonstrated to have the potential for the treatment of a wide variety of malignancies, and researchers are continuously working to create and perfect these treatments.

Precision medicine is a method of providing medical care that takes into consideration the genetic makeup, environmental circumstances, and lifestyle choices of a patient in order to devise individualized treatment plans for that patient. Precision medicine may be utilized in the field of immunology to locate particular genetic markers associated with the immune system that is amenable to being treated by various treatments. Research on the microbiome has proven that the microbiome of the gut, which is the collection of bacteria and other microorganisms that dwell in our digestive tract, has a crucial role in the function of the immune system. Researchers are continuing their investigations into the ways in which the microbiome and the immune system interact with one another, as well as the potential applications of these relationships for enhancing immune function.

Editing of genes: Technologies for editing genes, such as CRISPR-Cas9, have the potential to transform the field of immunology by enabling researchers to accurately edit the genomes of immune cells. This could be a game-changer for the field. This technology has the potential to be utilized in the development of new treatments for diseases and disorders connected to the immune system.

Understanding through computers and artificial intelligence: The study of immunology is benefiting from the application of artificial intelligence and machine learning technologies, which are assisting researchers in locating potential novel therapeutic targets and developing individualized treatment plans. These technologies could also be used to evaluate enormous datasets containing information relevant to the immune system in order to discover new patterns and insights.

The field of immunology has a promising future in general, and the current research that is being conducted in these and other areas holds promise for the future development of new treatments and therapies for immune-related diseases and disorders.

Conclusion

The Value of Having Immune to Disease

Immunity is critical to the continued existence of all living species, including humans, and their overall health and well-being. The following is a list of some of the important reasons why immunity is so crucial:

Defense against the spread of infection: The immune system is one of the most important defense mechanisms that the body possesses in its fight against infectious diseases. It is tasked with recognizing foreign pathogens, including viruses, bacteria, and parasites, and eliminating them from the body once discovered. Keeping one's health and one's well-being in check: Having a robust immune system can help improve overall health and well-being as well as the prevention of chronic diseases. It is necessary for the body to function correctly and to defend itself against potential dangers.

The reaction to the injury: In addition, the immune system is engaged in the process by which the body reacts to injuries and stress. It promotes healing and regeneration, assists in the removal of damaged cells and tissues, and helps clear away damaged cells and tissues.

Vaccine research and development: The study of immunity has resulted in the creation of vaccinations, which have been essential in preventing infectious diseases that were formerly major dangers to public health. Vaccines have also been helpful in reducing the number of deaths caused by infectious diseases.

Regarding the therapy of diseases: Recent developments in the scientific discipline of immunology have resulted in the creation of innovative treatments and therapies for a wide range of ailments, including cancer and autoimmune disorders.

In general, immunity is necessary for the continued existence and health of all living species, and it is a vital field of research that has led to a number of significant discoveries and breakthroughs in the prevention and treatment of disease.

In this section, we will review the significance of the immune system to the health and well-being of humans.

The immune system is absolutely necessary for the health and well-being of a human being. A quick review of some of the essential reasons why immunity is so crucial is as follows: Defense against infection: the immune system is in charge of recognizing and eliminating invading pathogens, including viruses, bacteria, and parasites. This is how the immune system works to protect the body. This aids in the body's defense against diseases that are caused by infectious agents.

Keeping one's health and well-being in good standing requires one to have a robust immune system in order for the body to function appropriately and successfully fend off potential dangers. It can boost overall health and well-being in addition to assisting in the prevention of chronic diseases.

The immune system plays a role in the way the body reacts to injuries and trauma, and this includes the body's response to injuries. It promotes healing and regeneration, assists in the removal of damaged cells and tissues, and helps clear away damaged cells and tissues.

The study of immunity has led to the creation of vaccinations, which have been essential in preventing infectious diseases that were formerly serious dangers to public health. Vaccines have also played an important role in the management of existing immune responses.

Disease treatment: Recent developments in the scientific discipline of immunology have resulted in the creation of innovative treatments and therapies for a wide range of diseases, including cancer and autoimmune disorders.

In conclusion, immunity is very important to the health and well-being of humans, and the study of immunology has resulted in a great number of significant discoveries and breakthroughs in the prevention and treatment of disease. It is crucial for general health to have a robust immune system since this can assist in protecting against a wide range of dangers to our well-being and can help to prevent illness.

A rallying cry was supporting the maintenance of research and education efforts regarding immunity.

It is absolutely necessary for the continued health and well-being of individuals and populations all over the world for there to be continual study and education on immunity. The following are some of the reasons why we must maintain our investment in this sector:

The emergence of previously unknown diseases: The most recent COVID-19 pandemic serves as a sobering illustration of how rapidly new diseases can originate and spread across the globe. It is critical to maintain research efforts and educate people about immunity in order to improve our understanding of how to avoid and manage these diseases.

Rising prevalence of chronic diseases, the incidence of chronic diseases such as diabetes, cardiovascular disease, and cancer is increasing all across the world. Immune dysfunction is frequently associated with various disorders; therefore, ongoing research on immunity as well as education on the topic, are required in order to gain a deeper understanding of the underlying mechanisms and to create new treatments.

Population aging: There is a rising need to better understand how the immune system changes with age and how to promote healthy aging as the world's population ages. This is because the global population is getting older.

Continued study in this subject has the potential to uncover novel treatments and cures for some of the world's most serious health concerns, and it has already led to the development of new therapeutics for a wide range of diseases. Possibility for new therapies:

Knowing the immune system and how it reacts to infectious diseases is critical for both public health preparedness and response. Understanding the immune system is also important for public health preparedness. It is absolutely necessary to carry on research and teaching efforts pertaining to immunity in order to assist us in becoming better prepared for future disease outbreaks.

In a nutshell, we need to keep pouring money into studies and classes that focus on the immune system so that we may gain a deeper understanding of how it functions, how it can be strengthened, and how we can tap into its potential to ward off and treat illness. In order to guarantee that the positive outcomes of this research are distributed widely and fairly, it will be necessary to maintain funding, maintain collaboration, and engage the public.

www.ingramcontent.com/pod-product-compliance
Lightning Source LLC
Chambersburg PA
CBHW061605250726

48657CB00017B/1991